Cries

from the

Barren

Womb

Cries
from the
Barren
Womb

Julie Lortz

CROSSBOOKS
PUBLISHING

CrossBooks™
A Division of LifeWay
1663 Liberty Drive
Bloomington, IN 47403
www.crossbooks.com
Phone: 1-866-879-0502

First published by CrossBooks 04/24/2012

ISBN: 978-1-4627-1681-4 (sc)
ISBN: 978-1-4627-1682-1 (e)

Library of Congress Control Number: 2012906926

Printed in the United States of America

This book is printed on acid-free paper.

Contents

Chapter 1: It's So Bleak

"Lord, thank you that I don't have a child," I silently prayed as tears rolled down my cheeks. Even as I conveyed those simple words in a brief prayer, I couldn't believe that I not only said them but also truly meant them.

It was April 2010, and on that particular day and in that exact moment, the sharpness of a slightly misguided needle sent searing pain through my right leg. "That's not supposed to hurt," the specialist said. But it did.

Every muscle and joint in my body hurt. I could barely move. I needed help for normal everyday tasks. I wiped the tears from my face and whispered softly, "Oh, but it does." He patted my hand, smiled, and told me it was almost over. I had been down this road before. The difference that time was that I knew exactly what was wrong, and it was only a matter of time before the doctors realized it too. For the second time in my life, I found myself undergoing one medical test after another. But the emotion of what was to come was as painful as the physical torment ravaging my body.

As I lay on the table for the remainder of the test, I contemplated the gratefulness I felt for not having a child.

How did I get to that point? For years, I had cried until I had no tears left because I desperately wanted a child. I still do. Every time a friend had a baby, my heart hurt so badly I couldn't bear it. At different times throughout the years, I couldn't even bring myself to go to church. Yet here I was, thanking God for not fulfilling that desire. What in the world was going on? In that moment, I realized how far I had come in this heart-wrenching journey.

Perhaps you're reading this because you are on that same journey. Or perhaps you know someone who is. The experiences shared by women like me are universal. Maybe one of these scenarios sounds familiar:

> I hosted baby shower after baby shower, and
> with each one, I grew increasingly aware
> that while I spent hour after hour and dollar
> after dollar for someone else, I would never
> get to experience that elation myself. For
> so long I enjoyed it, but as I was preparing
> for a shower one afternoon, I realized the
> extreme emotional toll it had taken on my
> soul. I was decorating with the baby confetti
> they make for showers, and a couple pieces
> fell off the table. As I bent over to pick them
> up, huge tears fell on the tile. I couldn't stop
> them, and I did not want to. I sat down on
> the floor and wept. I didn't know what else
> to do. I knew then that I had hosted my
> last baby shower for the foreseeable future,
> perhaps forever.

People frequently assume that because I don't have children, I don't like them. Nothing could be further from the truth. Yet time and time again, I have found myself excluded from days in the park or a lunch get-together because I don't have a child. The reality of this exclusion is heartache piled on top of almost unbearable heartache.

I have been asked what is wrong with me more times than I can count—the perception being that not having a child makes me inferior to a woman who does. As if I didn't feel inadequate enough, having someone point out the obvious is another excruciating reminder of the "never going to happen."

Mother's Day celebrations were a yearly reminder of what would never be my reality. I couldn't bring myself to go to church, knowing there would be something to highlight those who were mothers and I would be left out. There is no special day or emphasis for the barren woman. There is only the silent cry from a womb that will never carry a child.

> I don't want others to feel like they have
> to walk on eggshells when they are around
> me, and I definitely don't want anyone to
> diminish the great gift of life. Yet I don't
> want to be demeaned or stepped on while
> they do. I've just wanted a little awareness,
> sensitivity, and dignity in the process.

The list could go on and on. The daily reminder of what would never be rang in my ears and permeated my thoughts. So how did I get to that point?

The word *barren* evokes in me a vision of a large, empty land with no water, no trees—a land essentially unfit for human habitation. I am mildly amused at the previous sentence because that's exactly what the situation is for women unable to conceive a child: our wombs are unfit for human habitation. Ten years ago, I wouldn't have found that the least bit witty, let alone have written it down on paper for the world to read. It hasn't always been that way.

I remember an incident that happened in a former workplace one day. I had two coworkers; one was a man, and the other a woman. I had worked for about a year with the man, and we were fairly familiar with each other. Shortly after the young woman started her employment, she revealed that she was pregnant. I recall thinking, "Oh, great, just what *I* need," as if it were all about me. I was at a place in my life where I really didn't even want to be around a pregnant woman, hear about a pregnant woman, or even think about pregnancy. Because everything in my life at that time was about me, it seemed that my needs and wants were most important. Over the course of the next few months, all she talked about was her baby. Day in and day out, I endured the tumultuous emotional roller coaster of listening to a play-by-play of what was happening to her physically, emotionally, and mentally, and it became far too much for me to bear. My demeanor toward her changed in such a way that I found myself a little hostile. One day, she was discussing the ultrasound she'd had that morning. It was the third or fourth time I had listened to the recitation. I was fed up. I got up and closed the door between our workstations … hard. Well, truth be told, I slammed the door. It was obvious to everyone it was not an accident. I was tired of all the baby talk and felt the need to be a baby about it myself.

Sadly, this is a pretty accurate picture of much of my behavior. Most of the ten years it took me to get to a place of acceptance were spent in tears and fits of rage, and heaven help me, pregnant woman after pregnant woman was left in my wake. Most of them probably didn't even know what had hit them, why it had hit them, or what they had done to deserve such treatment. There was clearly something wrong, and the reason they couldn't figure it out was because what was wrong was me. I was angry at God, sometimes furious. After all, He is the God of the universe and can create or change as He sees fit, so why not change this part of me? For so long, I had more questions than answers. At times it almost drove me crazy. There were seasons where I was honestly concerned for my own mental well-being. I am not one of those people who easily accepts the unknown or partially known. Everything has a reason, and eventually, those reasons should be revealed. God doesn't necessarily work that way. The truth is that many questions will never be answered this side of heaven. I've realized that I'm blessed to know the answers to some things, and for others, I have to trust God to do what is best for me.

There are many places in Scripture that point to this very thing—God appearing to not answer or delay the answer. Joseph comes to mind. I imagine he had more questions than answers as he was sold into slavery by his brothers, falsely accused by Potiphar's wife, and then thrown in prison for years. For a brief time, he thought he might get out, but once again, he was forgotten by those around him. There were days when it must have been incredibly difficult for him to cling to his faith and trust the One who knew the reasons. I wonder if there were times in that dark, damp prison cell that he thought he might lose his mind. Did he lose hope? Did he cry out in agony?

I think of Daniel being carried off to Babylon as a young man, never to set foot in his homeland again. He was taken into the king's service; he had to learn a different culture and live in a manner completely foreign to him. Did he despair of life? Or did he wonder what in the world was happening or how anything good could come from his circumstance?

Even in blessings, there may be questions that go unanswered. In 2 Samuel 7, we find the story of King David being settled in his palace and the Lord giving him rest from his enemies. David desired to build a temple to house the ark of God. Instead, the Lord told David through the prophet Nathan that He would build a house for David's household. Read 2 Samuel 7:18 and write David's questions below.

_____

_____

_____

_____

God had just established a covenant with David, and he could not understand why God would do that. Why him? Why that time? What on earth was God thinking? The truth is that there are so many questions that will go unanswered for us.

One day as I scoured over the Scriptures in search of stories about barren women, I came across a passage in Judges 13. This particular chapter is about the birth of Samson and the events preceding his birth.

What is the situation of Manoah and his wife in verse 2?

_____

_____

Who appears to Samson's mother in verse 3, and what does he promise?_____

_____

_____

The woman relayed this story to her husband, Manoah, who prayed and asked God to send the angel again to teach them how to raise this promised child. God heard

Julie Lortz

Manoah's prayer, and the angel visited his wife again. This time, she went to get her husband, and he came to speak to the angel. A brief conversation ensued between the angel and Manoah, and he asked the Lord to tell him His name.

What was the response of the angel of the Lord in verse 18?

_____

_____

_____

This simplicity of this answer speaks volumes to me: "It is beyond understanding" (Judges 13:18). Sometimes God doesn't answer our questions because the answer is beyond our human understanding. We don't think like God. We don't see the entire realm of eternity, so we really can't wrap our finite, human brains around His omniscient, eternal activities. Isaiah puts it this way: "For my thoughts are not your thoughts, neither are your ways my ways" (Isaiah 55:8).

This doesn't mean we can't ask God whatever we want. In fact, the opposite is quite true. God invites us to ask questions and go to Him with our deepest wounds. I present to you the psalms as evidence. Below are listed just a few examples. What questions do we see asked in these verses?

Psalm 6:3_____

_____

Psalm 10:1_____

_____

Psalm 13:1–2_____

_____

Psalm 22:1_____

_____

While God may invite us to ask questions, what we need to remember is that in spite of the answer or the lack of an answer, we must keep believing, trusting, and walking in faith.

There are many reasons why women find themselves in this situation—some by choice, others by nature of being single, some by illness or disease, others by an accident, some as a result of their husband's infertility, and still others by infertility as a result of their sinful choices early in life. Regardless of how we end up in this situation, I guarantee most feel a wide range of emotions as a result. Those who choose to be childless suffer because of the opinions of others who, rather than respect the women's decisions, constantly accuse them of selfishness or barrage them with questions and criticize their every move. Those like me who are barren by no choice of their own may suffer from sorrow, guilt, anger, resentment, and an ache in their soul that never seems to fade. We're also frequently asked the "why" questions. If only we had answers. I've met women over the years that aren't able to have children as the result of their husband's infertility. Rare (but oh-so-beautiful) is the woman who harbors no bitterness toward her husband as a result. Finally, there are women who are barren as a result of their own sinful choices. They suffer from guilt and never-ending "what if" questions.

God has taken me to the very depths of hurt and anger surrounding my inability to have children. To say I've spent season after season in a pit of despair over this situation is a precise, albeit sad statement. For ten years, God and I wrote my testimony on this subject, and in all honesty, it could have been a much shorter time, had I not fought Him with extreme intensity. Because of my own selfishness and sinfulness, the process lasted far too many years. Gratefully, God did not give up on me, and He did not allow Satan the victory. I have come out of this bruised, battered, and broken, but by the grace of God, I have emerged and bring with me a vision and assignment from God to help others in the same situation.

If you are one of these women, my prayer is that you find a few answers in this writing, but more than that, I hope you will ultimately find peace in the place where God has put you, even if the answers don't come. I do understand what you think and feel, and I have come to believe God has used this part of my life to encourage others and bring them to a place where they understand their value in Christ. Rest assured that you are not alone; even if you don't know another woman in your circumstance, God is always there. He does understand, and He desires that you accept His help to overcome what appears to be an insurmountable chasm.

If you are someone who loves a woman or couple in this situation, I hope to shed some light on the deep emotions and despair that can come with infertility. Perhaps you will find a few helpful hints to help you love them through this and lead them to Christ for help and hope.

Chapter 2: Chosen by God

To fully understand my perspective and the reasons behind writing this book, I think it is essential to give you some background on my family life, childhood, and the events leading up to my barrenness. I will also share with you stories of other women I have had the privilege of interviewing and getting to know through this process. I am certain their stories will bless and encourage you.

I grew up in a large family with two brothers and two sisters as well as a stepbrother and stepsister who were around frequently during those early years of my childhood. My mom came from an enormous family with ten children total, so we had relatives all over the place. My dad, however, came from a smaller family, just two sisters, and both of them lived out of state. We were a churchgoing family, and I made a decision to give my life to Christ when I was ten years old. I look back on my childhood and realize that it was truly idyllic. Our main job during those years was just to be kids. Don't get me wrong—we had chores to do and were given responsibility according to our ages; however, most of the time, we went to school and spent time with our friends. Our neighborhood was full of kids, and we were free to roam, to learn, and to discover the treasures kids find so valuable. We were allowed a safe, happy childhood where our innocence was protected and we were pointed to Christ.

Like most little girls, I had many dreams as I was growing up. Also like most little girls, those dreams varied from year to year and sometimes from day to day. Some days, I knew I would grow up and be a doctor, other days, I wanted to be a lawyer. Other days, I wasn't going to work but just travel. I had more ideas than I could ever fulfill in a lifetime. I remember in the fifth grade, we had an assignment to make a picture of something that reflected what we would do when we grew up. We went to the big rolls of paper, chose our color, and the teacher ripped off a large piece so we could cut out a shape and fill it in. I surveyed all the colors and knew immediately I would need brown. I had to make a desk. So I got to work, cut out part of the middle where my legs would go, and drew in the drawers, knobs, and handles. We each paraded ours in front of the class to hang them on the wall, and I proudly announced that the desk symbolized I would be a secretary! Until that day, the thought of being a secretary had never crossed my mind, and rarely after that day did it again; however, on that day I was certain.

No matter what dream I had about a job or career, house or travel, two things were always certain: I would be married (to the most handsome, romantic prince in the world), and I would have children. It never crossed my mind that my life might not have both of those things. I look back now and see those expectations as the beginning of my later disappointment. I had set expectations for myself without realizing they might not be in God's plan for my life. I've since learned that the greatest source of disappointment in my life is due to unrealistic expectations just like those. Sometimes I put them on myself, sometimes on other people, and sometimes they are put on me. In the end when I don't quite measure up or the person I have put the expectation on doesn't measure up, I'm left with nothing but disappointment. It's a vicious cycle that took me a long time to get out of so that I could continue on with realistic living.

About six months after I turned fifteen, unusual things began to happen to me. I went to a high school that was three levels, and as I climbed the stairs between my classes, sometimes I would fall. Of course everybody laughed. I felt stupid, made some sort of clumsy excuse, picked up my books, and went on. It became more frequent. Before long, it was hard for me to get out of bed in the morning. Later, I developed a rash on my right leg, left arm, chest, back, and face. So began a series of doctor visits that lasted over three months. Rarely did a week pass that I didn't receive a note in class saying my mom was waiting for me and I was excused. I was poked, prodded, and tested until my arms and legs ached. Each time they diagnosed me with something, my dad would research what vitamins and supplements were thought to help, and he would go to the health food store to stock up on my latest needs. He was desperate to do anything and everything to make life more bearable for me.

One day, I received a note in class and went out to meet my mom. As I got closer to the car, I noticed it was not my mom in the driver's seat but rather my dad. I was immediately seized by fear because my dad did not generally take time off work to go to the doctor with us. Mom just handled it, so I knew something was different this time. Something was definitely wrong. A sense of dread enveloped me as I trudged to the car. I got in the backseat and asked the usual question, "Where are we going today?"

My mom looked straight ahead, but my dad turned around and explained we were going to see a man named Dr. Smith. From recent testing, it appeared I had a disease called lupus. Up to that point, I had never heard of lupus and had no idea how horrible it was. Dad told me it was a very serious disease, and as I stared at him in disbelief, my eyes welled up with tears. His did, too. As he blinked back tears of his own, dad turned to face forward, and my mom turned around and said, "No matter what happens, we will do whatever it takes to get you the best medical attention there is." We drove the rest of the way in silence. It was only a couple of miles to the doctor's office, but it seemed like it took an eternity to get there. At the same time, however, we arrived all too soon. As we sat in the waiting room, I was filled with both dread and anticipation. The idea that we finally knew what we were dealing with was comforting, yet the possible outcome was too frightening to think about.

By God's grace, Dr. Smith was wrong that day. He sent me over for a muscle biopsy, and one week before my sixteenth birthday, the results came back. I had a form of muscular dystrophy in conjunction with rheumatoid arthritis. It is a disease that acts similar to lupus but is actually an inflammatory disease rather than a deteriorating one. While it may not sound like it, that was great news! From what one doctor told us, the two diseases actually kind of complemented each other, making neither as serious as they could be separately. We immediately began treatment. We went through a wide variety of medications, mixing and matching until we came up with the perfect combination. What seemed to work best was a medication that came with a whole host of its own problems; however, I was able to tolerate it better than most others, and the results were respectable.

Over the next four years, we worked toward the goal of reducing my medication to zero if possible. While there were up days and down days, we managed the disease successfully. I was slower at some things than most people but could continue the majority of my activities with additional effort. There was not a lot known about my disease at that time, and while we did not really know what to do and what not to do, my mom did the one thing she was convinced would help me. She was adamant that I keep moving. She was determined not to let me sit at home and wallow in self-pity. She had me walk with her after school, and depending on the day, we would walk a block or three miles. It all came down to how I was feeling at the time. One day in particular, she stopped, turned to me, and said, "Julie, I know you don't feel well, and I know it stinks. I know you don't think it's fair. Life is not fair. Sometimes we get handed things we don't understand. You can choose to let this disease make you bitter, or you can use the circumstances to make your life better."

I pondered that for a few moments, not quite sure what to make of it. It seemed pretty profound to that sixteen-year-old. As those ideas swirled through my head, her voice broke through my thoughts as she continued, "But as long as you live in my house, you will not be bitter and make the rest of us miserable. Do what you need to do to deal with it and then get on with your life."

At the time, I thought it was cruel and, quite frankly, rude. In hindsight, however, that was a pivotal point in that journey as well as so many others after that. What she said is absolutely true. Life is not fair. Things happen to us that we don't like and that we certainly did not ask for, and if given the choice, we would say "no thanks" to most of these instances. We frequently don't get that choice. My mom taught me a lesson that day I would never forget—a lesson that would help me so much throughout my life.

It was also during this time that I met the man who is now my husband. One day, we were hiking in the mountains, and I was completely exhausted. I suddenly realized the impact this would have on the rest of my life, and I didn't think I would ever find somebody who would be willing to deal with my limitations. Within seconds, I was plummeting to an all-out pity party. At this point, I had no idea the impact on my life included not having children. Steve asked me if I wanted to sit down to rest, and I did everything I could to hold the tears back. He asked what was wrong, and I put it all out there. I told him everything. I expected that to be our last outing together, but instead, he looked at me and said words I will never forget. He allowed me to finish my thoughts, and then he did not hesitate before he spoke the following words: "Did you ever think maybe that's why God brought me into your life?" To understand the enormity of this wisdom, it might help you to be aware of the fact that he was only seventeen at the time. I knew from that day forward we would get married one day, but I had no idea it would be a short two years later on June 24, 1988, when I was barely twenty years old.

Once married, I joined Steve in Phoenix, where he was going to college. Both of us had grown up in the church and understood (at least conceptually) the value of consistent fellowship, teaching, and spiritual growth. Still dealing with the death of his mother when he was just sixteen, Steve had not found a church to attend in the previous nine months. Even though he didn't realize it at the time, the reason was because he was dealing with the same emotions I was wrestling with but for different reasons. He had unmet expectations and unanswered questions from God. Once I arrived, we did not make it a priority to do so either. As a matter of fact, I found a job in retail, and that became our reason for not being able to go to church. We did not really want to attend, but it was easier for our consciences if we had what we perceived as a legitimate reason. We began down a road of self-reliance that set the stage for an out-of-control downward spiritual spiral.

Almost two years into our marriage, it became apparent I would not be able to use the birth control pill in the long term. As I spoke to my doctor about other options, he said the pill was the most reliable, and while I could use other forms of birth control, the chance of pregnancy increased. He went on to say that I really shouldn't have a child while on the medication for my disease because of the severe birth defects and high risk of retardation in a fetus. They also had no idea what would happen to my body under the strain and stress of pregnancy and childbirth. I could have seen anything from minor inconveniences to total debilitation. We were not prepared to deal with any of those problems. I was shocked to hear him say these words: "If you do get pregnant, abortion is another form of control." I was flabbergasted! Abortion was never going to be an option for me, and I didn't hesitate to tell him so. He said the risks were too high, that we should never attempt a pregnancy, and finally, he recommended a surgical option. We conceded, but I have to admit I was not prepared for the emotional aftermath. I pretended it didn't exist. I plunged headlong into years of denial. My initial denial came because, medically speaking, I still had every internal organ required to give birth, so it was not real to me. In my mind, I had fixed the problem of birth control, and while I knew it was permanent, I did not fully allow myself to accept that concept. I could change it anytime I wanted to and had every intention of doing so. But God had a different plan, and these years of denial and disbelief would end up pushing me over the edge.

In the midst of this ordeal, a most amazing blessing was granted to my family. It was February 23, 1990, and a beautiful baby girl was born to my sister. It was years before cell phones and digital cameras, and I could barely wait for the first picture to arrive in the mail. Every day I anxiously looked in the mailbox, and on the days Steve picked me up from work, my first question was whether or not the photo had arrived. At last it did, and I held on to that picture as if I were holding on for dear life. Even though separated by many miles and many states, that precious baby became one of the great loves of my life. Erica Lorraine was such a joy to me in the midst of my despair and darkness. I cherished every picture, letter, and phone conversation. Each visit was a treasure to me. I ached to hold her, and when given the chance to wrap that precious baby in my arms, I never wanted to let her go. She still means the world to both me and Steve.

In June 1991, a year and a half later, Steve went to Officer Candidate School for the US Marine Corps, and that fall, we moved to Virginia. Six months later, we migrated to North Carolina. I was still in the ups and downs of my disease, but it was soon discovered that there was a possible connection between my disease and female hormones. My rheumatologist referred me to a gynecologist who did a series of tests. His findings were vague to say the least. He basically said that while they could not link the two definitively, there was strong evidence to suggest they were indeed linked. How do you like that? If they couldn't make heads or tails of it, how was I supposed to? After much discussion between the two of them and me and Steve, we came to the conclusion that the best option was a hysterectomy. It was scheduled for January 7, 1994, and I was twenty-five years old.

A week after the surgery, Steve went out on his scheduled, three-month deployment, and I was completely alone, totally ill-equipped for the roller-coaster ride I was about to experience. He was part of the advance party going to the military exercises, so he left a week before the majority of his squadron. The following weekend was a four-day holiday weekend, so most of the people I knew went away or spent family time with their husbands before they shipped out too. It was the longest weekend I have ever had in my life. The neighborhood was practically empty. There was nothing on television, and I was homebound, unable to drive and barely able to walk.

Looking back, I see God was trying desperately to reach out to me; however, it had been several years since I had been in close relationship with Him, and I was not interested. In my mind, the entire situation from the disease to the hysterectomy was His fault. I grew up listening to the stories of how powerful God was and how everything was subject to Him. At any point, He could have healed me of my disease, completely restored my health, and enabled me to have children. And yet He did not do any of those things. His plan was for complete restoration but not physical healing. There I was in North Carolina, my husband in California, my family in Montana and Minnesota, and I had no church family. I resolved my loneliness problem promptly the following Monday morning by calling the cable company and getting cable television installed. It worked for a while, and I was temporarily able to drown the voice of God with the television running almost twenty-four hours a day. It is intriguing that when things happened I did not like,

I easily and readily blamed God. Yet as the good things happened early in our marriage, I attributed it to how hard we had worked and the efforts we had put in. Had I been paying attention, I would have recognized these instances as huge markers of our spiritual decline.

My healing time after the hysterectomy was extended because of the other medical problems I had, and the intensity of my disease increased during this time. This was the darkest time in my life up to this point. In retrospect, it continues to be one of the darkest, mainly because I had no hope. Even though my first surgery had been three and a half years earlier, I had not dealt with the emotions or allowed God to heal me. As mentioned earlier, I knew at the time the operation was permanent, but I had always hoped in the back of my mind that we could work around that. All of a sudden, I knew it was real. My life had moved down a one-way street, and there was no way back to change things, even though I desperately wanted to do so.

While Steve was gone for ten weeks, I decided I knew exactly what he was thinking and that he would eventually leave me to find a woman who could give him a family. I did not bother to ask him what he thought. I just decided I knew. I put much thought into how I would broach the subject when he returned. I played conversation after conversation in my head, and in each instance, I really believed I was doing him a favor by offering him a way out. When he returned, I picked a time and stupidly told him he was free to go, because I knew he would leave me eventually anyway and it was better sooner than later. This way, he could still find somebody while he was young and start a family. I will never forget the look on his face. It is seared into my memory forever. I'm not sure if I would describe it as a look of horror, a look of disappointment, or a look of disbelief. Maybe it was a combination of all three. I will also never forget the words he said before he turned and walked into the garage. He said, "You just don't get it, do you? If you can't have kids, I can't have kids, because it isn't about you or me. It's about us. If it happens to you, it happens to me. We're in this together. Till death do us part." In my self-pity I had completely underestimated his commitment to and his love for me. I basically told him I did not trust or believe him, and the words I said cut deep to his soul. Even at the time, I realized the sadness. By playing out this scenario, I led our marriage down a path that led us to a place requiring years of work to fix.

At this particular place in the story, I feel the need to stop and say a word to those women who may have experienced the trauma caused by a husband who chose not to honor the wedding vows and moved on in the end. While I cannot speak to this firsthand, I can imagine the horror, because I rehearsed it in my head countless times. In the end, I know that God is faithful, and I can guarantee that He is still by your side. His promise in Joshua 1:5 is quite clear: "I will never leave you nor forsake you." No matter what choices other people make, God will still make something beautiful out of a life surrendered to Him. Run directly to Him and receive the comfort that only He can provide.

I'm not sure I can fully explain every emotion I experienced, but I can tell you it was everything from fear to sorrow to guilt to anger to depression to resentment to self-pity. On the positive side, four months after surgery, my disease went into remission. I don't know that I fully appreciated it at that time, but in the years that followed, I certainly did. I enjoyed that remission until November 2009.

Many years have passed since that bleak January in 1994, but I still vividly recall everything I went through and everything I felt. This event was not the end of our sorrow. At the time, I could not have imagined things getting worse, but that was exactly what happened. Because of our rebellion and continuing refusal to align our lives with what God had planned for us, He continued to remove material things from us, and in March 1995, we found ourselves moving back to Montana, completely broken emotionally, physically, and spiritually. We weren't financially depleted, but that soon followed. We were at the bottom of the proverbial pit. In spite of all this brokenness, it took another year for us to realize our predicament was the result of seven years of poor choices, seven years of rebellion.

The following May, we finally returned to the home church we had grown up in and been married in. We had purposely stayed away because we were too proud. In our own minds, we had failed. To my surprise, we were welcomed back just like the prodigal son in Luke 15. They loved us, encouraged us, and gently restored us to the right relationship with God.

On August 22, 1997, another beautiful miracle came into our family. Peter Jerome Lyle, an amazingly tough, premature boy stormed our world. While completely different from his seven-year-old sister, he stole our hearts and won our affection just as easily. You will never meet a more tender-hearted boy. This time around, my sister and I lived in the same town, and I got to hold Peter whenever I wanted. I reveled in babysitting him and knowing everything about him firsthand. I was able to attend birthday parties, baseball games, church programs, and school award ceremonies. His birth caused me to take a serious look at my life and where I was headed. I was filled with anger, resentment, and bitterness. I knew if I wanted to have a positive impact on these children, I would have to let go and get spiritually healthy.

However, it wasn't until 1999 that I became determined enough to do the hard work required to get out of my rut. I tried everything from godly counseling to Bible studies and self-will. It all failed because I neglected to go to the source—God Himself. I had to confess that anger, resentment, and bitterness. I had to get serious with God and admit to myself that my focus was misplaced. The process was still quite long, even after that. There was layer after layer that caused my heart to be hard and calloused. Don't get me wrong. I grew in leaps and bounds in other areas of my spiritual life, and God used me; however, I was holding back this one part of my life, the part where my barrenness had defined who I was. It was too painful to relive and incredibly difficult to relinquish control, but I knew God was calling me to deal with this. And until I did, my growth would stop. I would be like the Israelites wandering in the desert for forty years. It was always easy for me to read about them and wonder how they could be so blind to what God was doing, and yet I had been walking in the same circle for ten long years. That happened in the fall of 2004, just four short months before I began journaling my thoughts, which have become the source of this writing. I began to write these words for myself to help process what had happened and was continuing to happen to me. Even then God had a bigger plan for what I had gone through, what I was currently going through, and what I would experience in the future. He had a magnificent plan for my story.

It's too soon for me to know all God's purposes surrounding my infertility. I may never know all of them this side of eternity. As I put the finishing touches on this work, I realized that it had been almost seven years since I had begun writing. Our lives have been on an amazing ride with God, including Steve's year-long deployment to Iraq, seeing God's unlimited comfort in the loss of my dad, a call on our lives to full-time ministry, and the resurgence of my muscular dystrophy and rheumatoid arthritis, this time far more severe than the first bout all those years ago. In that time, God has revealed to me several instances where not having a child has been a blessing for us. I have a hunch the best is yet to be seen. Perhaps the reason we could not have biological children is because God intends for us to be the parents of spiritual children in the ministry He has called us to, or maybe He intends to use me to encourage and uplift others in the same situation. Whatever the reason, I am confident He has my best interests at heart. And whatever happens, He'll get the glory, and I'll be just fine.

Oh, yes, it's been an insanely long journey, a road that has threatened my relationships, spiritual life, mental well-being, and emotional stability. Through it all, God's handiwork is evident. His fingerprints are everywhere, and He has purposed something so amazing for me I can barely believe it myself. But that is our God, the one who knows what is best for us and gives us the grace to deal with those things we never thought we could.

What is your story? Before I share the incredible stories of ministry friends and partners, I would like for you to begin journaling a few thoughts about events, people, and your relationship with God. Here are a few questions to get you started:

What are my circumstances? How do I feel about them? Who is on this journey with me? What part do they play?

_____

_____

_____

_____

_____

_____

_____

_____

_____

_____

_____

_____

_____

_____

_____

_____

_____

_____

_____

_____

_____

_____

_____

_____

_____

_____

_____

_____

_____

_____

_____

_____

Chapter 3: Love from across the Ocean

"For I know the plans I have for you," declares the Lord, "plans to prosper you and not to harm you, plans to give you a hope and a future."
—Jeremiah 29:11

WHEN TOM AND KELLY SAID their marriage vows on April 29, 1989, they had no idea that the verse they had chosen would come to life in a way they had never expected. Would they embrace the plans God had for their lives or try in vain with much heartache to pursue the plans they wanted?

Tom grew up in a family with five siblings, and while he always wanted children of his own, he didn't particularly care how many. Kelly grew up in a home with two siblings, and she always wanted to have a lot of children. Like so many of us, it never occurred to them when they married that the hopes and desires they held close would never become reality.

The Humphreys spent their first four years of marriage enjoying their time as a couple. They decided to start trying to get pregnant after that fourth year, and it wasn't until their third year of trying that they began fertility testing. Initially, the doctors found uterine scarring that theoretically wouldn't prevent a pregnancy but could have led to complications during pregnancy or miscarriage. Kelly had surgery to resolve that problem, but they were still unable to conceive. They were never told they were infertile; there was no real medical reason they could not have children of their own.

Tom and Kelly made the decision to begin using fertility drugs in a cyclical manner. They used them for a year and then took six months off because the emotional toll of not getting pregnant became too much for Kelly. They continued that cycle for four years. Their next alternative was in vitro fertilization. They ruled this option out fairly early for a number of reasons. First, it was extremely expensive. Second, there were no guarantees, but most importantly, they saw this as a moral issue because of their firm belief that life began at the point of conception. The fate of the unused embryos was of paramount importance to them.

For the first few years of their infertility battle, they had a group of friends who were all in a similar life stage. The friendships grew and blossomed, and as always happens, they began, couple by couple, having child after child. Besides the Humphreys, there were one or two other couples experiencing the same struggles. Some of them withdrew from the group, whereas Kelly acted as if it were not a problem. After get-togethers, she would go home and cry. She was angry, frustrated, and sad, yet she hosted baby shower after baby shower because she did not want to rob others of their joy. She felt it was expected of her, and Kelly tended to be a people pleaser.

Early in the process, Tom brought up adoption, something he was passionate about, but Kelly was not open to the idea. He backed off, believing that if it was in God's plan for their lives, He would work on Kelly's heart at some point in the future.

As I spoke with these dear friends of mine, the stories they told and feelings they expressed were a page out of my own life. If I had not been looking at their faces as they spoke, I would have sworn it was a conversation taking place in my own head. I know many others in this situation can relate to them as well. One of their friends had a child already and was in complete turmoil because she couldn't have "just one more." She thought Tom and Kelly should understand how that feels, but for a childless couple, there is no understanding. They wanted even just one and would have been content with that. No, they could not comprehend that statement.

Here's what Tom told me: "They (friends) think they are trying to protect you by not including you in birthday parties and days in the park, but they don't understand how badly they are really hurting you by doing this. Others have no idea what to do. The truth is there is no cookie-cutter answer as to what should be done. It varies based on the couple. The key is to acknowledge the hurt and that you can't fix it. Please don't say you understand, particularly when you have a child you tuck in every night."

For Kelly, putting on a front made her feel okay as doing so caused her to be included. It allowed other couples to talk to her, but inside, she was slowly dying. She would frequently exclaim to Tom, "I can't do it anymore!" Her predicament was this: She did not want to be so fragile that if somebody said "baby" around her, she would crumble. She did not want to steal their happiness and joy. Yet she didn't want to spend the entire social event discussing pregnancy, childbirth, and child-rearing. Yes, talk about it but then move on to a conversation that includes everyone.

Does that resonate with anyone else besides me?

As I listened to them talk, there was further confirmation that what I am doing in this book is important and valuable. It is something God intended for me to do. Kelly expressed things I felt too, so I know we are not alone in this. She felt as if she were all alone, that nobody would want to listen, and even if they did, they would not understand. It wasn't until she met others with this same problem that she ceased feeling like something was wrong with her.

In 1995, the Humphreys moved to Montana because of Tom's job. They soon found a doctor specializing in infertility and continued the treatments. Finally, in 1999, the doctor said, "I can't do anything more for you until you go to a fertility clinic out of the state. Or you can adopt." Those words sent Kelly sobbing to a friend's house. It was over. It had actually been over years earlier, but to hear a doctor say it made it real. She was inconsolable.

Through their entire pursuit of fertility issues, Tom was the realist. He was the stronger of the two, and by her own admission, Kelly was a wreck. Most of the emotion Tom felt stemmed from Kelly's turmoil, doubt, and questioning. He couldn't fix it. By nature, Tom is a problem solver and fixer. However, in this situation, there was nothing he could do. Yet through it all, he felt there were other ways to have a family.

They finally made the decision to stop using fertility drugs. It had become too great a burden for Kelly to bear; the emotional toll was too much. Their resolve became this: "If God wants us to have children, we will in His time and in His way."

Again, Tom brought up adoption. Years earlier, as a new believer, he had read an article about the one-child-policy in China. It broke his heart. Through that article, God planted a seed in his heart, and Tom knew that at some point, he would adopt a child from China. He just didn't know it would be in lieu of a biological child.

They went to classes about stateside adoption. The agency was firm in their resolve that it be an open adoption. It was during the same time when stories permeated the news about parents who had given up their children, but who had had a change of heart, had come back for custody and torn apart established families. Tom and Kelly did not believe that such a situation would offer a stable environment in which to raise a child and there would be confusion and conflict over authority and parenting decisions. To them, it was for the betterment of the child not to pursue that option.

Tom and Kelly sent away for information about international adoptions, specifically in China. At last, the paperwork arrived, and a mountain of paperwork it was. They found the process intimidating, even invasive. While they understood the value for the child, they soon discovered the physical, emotional, and financial toll it could take on a person, a couple, and their marriage. Tom completed the paperwork early on, but it took almost a year for Kelly to complete her portion. A year after they had received the packet, they sent their paperwork in. Then the waiting began. It took another year, bringing the total to two years, for their beautiful baby girl, Tally.

They did not choose Tally specifically. They answered questions about the health and age of the baby. They chose "healthy" and "infant to twelve months." Once matched with a child, it took a month for the travel documents, arrangements, last-minute forms, etc. At last, the day arrived, and Kelly got on a plane with her parents because they wanted her parents to be a huge part of the process. Tom stayed home so he could take time off once the baby arrived at their home.

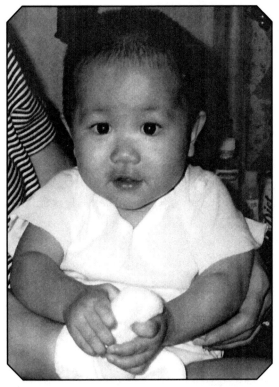

The story of sweet Tally is as amazing as it is heart-wrenching. She was abandoned as a newborn infant on a busy street corner in the city. She was found by a policeman and taken to an orphanage. Mothers did that intentionally, as they knew their child would be found. They hid so they could watch the child being picked up. Kelly and her parents were on the ground in China when Tally was eleven months old.

The new family returned home and remained a family of three for two and a half years. Tom thought it was important to pay back the money they had borrowed from family before they pursued another child. They knew the entire time they wanted to adopt again. They again chose China, but this time, they did so not only because of their soft hearts for that country but also because they wanted the siblings to have a common bond in their heritage and culture. They didn't want them to feel odd or unusual.

The second round of paperwork went faster, half the time, as they only had to add on to their portfolio. This time, Tom, Kelly, Tally, and Kelly's parents flew to China.

Teddi was ten months old when they landed on the ground. Her story is also a heartbreaker, as she was left at the orphanage door as a newborn infant, umbilical cord still attached. She was discovered in the morning by the director. She spent the entire ten months in that same orphanage before she was matched with the Humphreys.

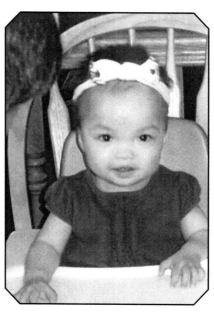

You will never meet two more different girls. Tally is very matter-of-fact. She acknowledges things, deals with them, and moves on. She is logical. She is a relational connecter. It is not uncommon for her to say, "I'm like my dad." As you might imagine, Tom just beams. Teddi is a tender, emotional six-year-old who internalizes everything. She is intuitive with the emotional side of life, which urges Tom and Kelly to protect her a little more. She feels and hurts deeply. Yet they comprise this beautiful family, one put together by God for a greater purpose in this part of the kingdom calendar.

The decision not to adopt again was not an easy one at which to arrive. While they would have considered it previously, the wait time for a child in China went from three to four to five years, and Tom and Kelly factored in their own ages as well. I wondered aloud about whether or not they had any regrets. Kelly's only one was that she waited so long to come around to adoption, but she felt to adopt in those emotional circumstances would not have been fair to a child. For Tom, however, there are no regrets, as he would not have the two girls he has. He sees this all as part of God's plan.

As one talks to Tom, the love and passion for his girls who were born in China is evident. His heart is so tender in regards to their culture and their journey into the lives of their American parents. He gets teary-eyed even talking about it. He is quick to tell them that they have an amazing story God will use in their lives. They are a true gift, part of a greater plan in the lives of Tom and Kelly and both will have a powerful voice enabling them to speak about adoption and orphanages as they grow into adulthood. God will gain much glory from their stories and already has a beautifully crafted plan for each one of these girls.

"Adoption is a beautiful process," Tom says. "It is a gift God put in our lives. It has been tangible evidence of God and His involvement in our lives and in the world."

Kelly adds, "The experience God let us have, to be able to go to a different country and to do this, is not something everybody gets to do. It's an awesome experience to pick up a beautiful child in another country."

When asked if they can give any advice, Kelly said, "That is so hard. To be on this side and try to tell somebody just starting that it's going to be okay is difficult. It's really only a relationship with the Lord that will fulfill that need, regardless of the end result. It can be adoption or perhaps no child at all." She has finally come to peace with the fact that her dream of a family of four biological children will never be a reality. She loves her family of two beautiful, international daughters. Even as she is ecstatic about her girls, at complete peace and wouldn't want it any other way, the simple fact is that sometimes it still hurts. When she finds herself in a conversation where each woman is talking about her pregnancy or childbirth, she feels an empty space. But with her journey, she knows she can help other women who feel the same way. That is one of the rewards a woman with a child can never experience.

Through all the things they experienced in their lives, God's plan became evident in the end, and Tom cannot imagine a more fulfilling plan in their lives. Their family is a real-life example of how Jeremiah 29:11 plays out. Rather than focus on the problem, Tom focused on what God's plan could be. He emphatically states, "It is all for His glory and good purpose. To the end, His kingdom will be glorified, and it's up to us to find ways to participate in that. It is not my job to create the plan, but it is my job to respond to the plan God has for my life." As they look back on their journey, they wish they would have reflected on that more often.

Interestingly, if you look at and evaluate the Humphrey family, Tally is a carbon copy of Tom. Teddi is a carbon copy of Kelly. Only God could have looked down from heaven and put the pieces in place for this culturally mixed family. It is a beautiful design that came out of a twelve year, heart-wrenching struggle with infertility. This family blesses my heart and gives encouragement to the many others longing for and desperately waiting for a child.

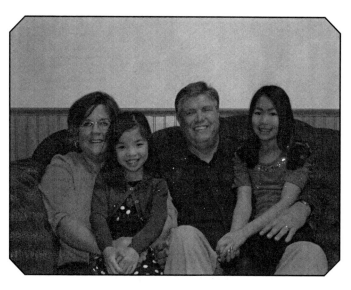

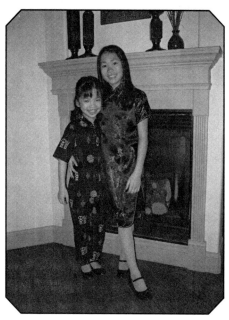

Chapter 4: The Waiting

I LOVE THE STORIES OF each person I interviewed. They are all friends of mine and have played profound roles in my life. I would not say that I am most excited about this story, particularly not over the others; however, because of timing, this story has taken a most interesting turn in the past few weeks, and I cannot help but want to jump out of my skin as I type.

Meet Michael and Christina, two of my colaborers in ministry. They have been married since 2005 and have worked in some sort of ministry that entire time. I've known or at least known of Michael since my teenage years. His family went to church with mine. Michael has one sister, and he moved around quite a bit until he was seven years old. It was then that his dad was transferred to Montana, where he spent the rest of his growing-up years here. Initially, they had no family close to them. They all lived in Texas, and the family made frequent trips to visit.

Michael's dreams are what I would term "guy dreams," meaning he was not nearly as detailed and romantic about them. He knew he wanted to go to college but never had anything specific in mind. He also knew he wanted to get married. He loved kids when he was growing up and worked with kids while he was in high school. He always assumed he'd have children of his own, three maximum. (His love of kids is something he's never lost. He is the elementary director at the church we both attend.)

Christina's background is quite different. She grew up with two sisters in Florida, and unlike Michael, she was surrounded by family—grandparents, aunts, uncles, and cousins were part of her everyday existence. She always wanted to get married and have children, a minimum of three. Note the irony of this pair! Strangely, even at a young age, she wondered what would happen if she could not have a child of her own.

These two met while in seminary in North Carolina, both already knowing they were called to ministry, specifically in Montana. Once married, they agreed to wait a year before they started a family, but at nine months, they decided they did not want to wait any longer. About three years into the marriage and after two years of trying to conceive, they knew there was a problem, but because they were in the middle of moving, they decided to wait until they settled in their new home to seek medical help.

They began the process of learning their options for testing, but before a single test was performed on Christina, it was discovered that Michael would not be able to father a child. They saw no need to continue testing because at that point, it did not matter. The reality was they would not have a child of their own. The reason this was particularly interesting to me is because prior to discussing this with Michael and Christina, every couple I had met where the husband was infertile, the wife had expressed anger and blame towards her husband. I had almost convinced myself that this was true in every situation like this. I could hardly wait for them to answer my next couple questions:

1. How did she feel? Without wavering, Christina emphatically stated that because she was never tested, they didn't know for certain what her results would have been. Nor would it have mattered.

2. I then asked, "Was there anger or blame?" A tear rolled down her cheek, and she slowly shook her head back and forth. "No, not for a second." Blaming never crossed her mind. She was not angry or upset, but rather her main concern was for Michael's mental and emotional well-being. She knew the responsibility he felt was tremendous, and her heart broke at the thought. For Christina, it was never a him-or-her situation. This was an issue for them as a couple, and it was something they would face together.

These amazing friends of mine shattered my very misplaced theory. There was no more evidence of marital strain in their marriage than in any other marriage I've ever witnessed. I secretly wondered to myself if I would have shown as much character and supportiveness had my situation taken this turn. With my mind already swarming, I nearly fell into a pile of tears as Michael continued with his own version.

He told me he had been praying that if there were a medical problem preventing them from having a child, it would be his. He felt he would be able to handle the news and would rather have that burden, regardless of his feelings, because he wanted to protect Christina. He did not want her to have to bear the sorrow and feelings of inadequacy that frequently accompany knowing it was an issue with you specifically. Whether those feelings make sense or not, I can testify that they are all too real. In the big scheme of God's plan for our lives, He is ultimately in control of that, but in an out-of-control, emotional situation, it takes a while to come to that understanding.

For the next several seconds, I stared almost in disbelief at Michael's face as he finished his thoughts. It's not that I thought he was being untruthful. I absolutely knew he was not. I was just so overcome with his vulnerability and his complete, unwavering commitment to and concern for his bride of five years. There was nothing but sheer genuineness in his words and his eyes. I will never forget it.

As is the case with every person I have ever met dealing with this issue, a mourning process ensued. No matter how the situation becomes a reality, it is a loss that must be faced, so mourning is normal. Even in the midst of this process, they rather quickly began looking into adoption options because prior to marriage, they had discussed and agreed upon the idea that they would have children of their own and adopt children. For Christina, much of her mourning came far later. As a matter of fact, it was in the spring of 2010, a story I will share with you in detail later.

Not wanting to let emotions get the better of them, they both acknowledged the struggles early on. Christina felt then, and still knows for certain that God has been very gracious to her. She has not been bitter when family and friends shared with her they were pregnant or when they had a baby. But it was hard just the same. About a year ago a mutual friend of ours was having a baby and we had both been invited to the shower. She called and asked me to be her "support buddy" at the shower. Even now that makes me smile. She did not want to rob our friend of the joy she was experiencing yet she knew going to the shower was going to be emotionally difficult for her. She did the one thing that guaranteed success: she admitted the pain and asked for help. There is no shame in that.

Christina admits she was plagued with the same questions many of us just like her have asked: Why do those who don't want children get to have them? Why is it so easy for some and so difficult for others? Michael concurred. "It seems unfair," he told me. "Maybe more than *seeming* unfair, it *is* unfair. Children are supposed to be a reward of waiting until you are married, and then when it doesn't happen, it throws you for a loop.

For a time, it feels like everything you've been taught is a lie."

My heart got heavy as I heard him say those words out loud. He put is so succinctly, so beautifully. Sadly, I think this is true on so many levels of our walk with Christ, particularly for those of us who grow up in the church. Somewhere along the line, we are led to believe that when we follow Christ, bad things will not happen to us. When a person grows up in Sunday school hearing about Daniel in the lion's den or David and his mighty men, we get the idea, whether created in our little minds or said outright by a teacher, that all the stories have perfectly happy endings. It is simply not true, and Scripture has just as many stories of defeat as victory. God does not promise that everything will work out as we think it should or as we would like. But He does promise that He will work all things together for God for those who love Him as are called according to His purpose. (See Romans 8:28.) I submit to you the story of Job as evidence that we can be upright and righteous yet still suffer much loss and hardship. Furthermore, Jesus told us in John 16:33 that we would have trouble. This should not surprise us. But there is great hope, as Jesus went on to tell us that He had overcome the world!

Early on, God gave Christina two thoughts that sustained her and helped obliterate the idea that we as believers should have it easier in this life. First, God took her to Matthew 5:45, "He causes His sun to rise on the evil and the good, and sends rain on the righteous and the unrighteous." Having children is part of God's "common grace" for all mankind. It is not specifically reserved for those who love Him and have given their lives to Him. Sin affects everything, including our bodies. Second, as salvation is a gift we are not worthy of receiving or one that we can attain through deeds, a child is a gift in the same kind of way. A person does not deserve it and cannot be good enough to achieve it. Life is a gift from God, and as such, the giver decides who gets that gift. It is not a payment for working hard or living right.

While they worked through all the emotions and took their options into account, they chose stateside adoption. International adoption was far too expensive for them to consider, and they almost immediately ruled out state adoption because the process included a foster-parent situation. Neither one of them felt it was in their best emotional interests to run the risk of having to return a child to the parent. They chose to go with a private agency, basing their decision mainly on the fact that their responses were quick and complete. They felt the initial interaction time would represent the rest of the process well. Having sent in the informational application, they received the second application, which included references and more detailed information and required a two-hundred-dollar application fee. They took a step of faith and sent it in only to discover the afternoon of that very day that Christina was getting a bonus. She was handed an envelope with exactly two hundred dollars in cash! It gives me goose bumps to hear that kind of story. They took that as confirmation that

God was indeed directing them to that exact agency to adopt a child.

Michael and Christina were invited to a weekend-long workshop; however, by that time, they experienced some turmoil in their lives, and they began to question whether or not it was a good idea to adopt a child. They were in the midst of extremely difficult season of ministry, wondering if they would even continue in full-time ministry. Adding to all this chaos, they easily came up with a list of reasons not to continue:

1. They had to do paperwork for the state as this was technically a foster-parent situation for the first six months. (Remember that this was one of their deciding factors that led them to a private agency.) While in the process, the state agency was revamping the paperwork, so they had additional paperwork all the time.

2. Continuing education was required to keep their foster-care license current. It was renewable every year.

3. The paperwork was extremely invasive and personal. This is the exact thing I had heard from Tom and Kelly in the previous chapter.

4. There was even more paperwork specific to the agency because they only did open adoptions, meaning the birth mother got to

review profiles and choose the prospective parents. They also encouraged an ongoing relationship with the birth mother if she desired that. This paperwork included twelve more single-spaced pages of questions for them to answer—questions about family relationships, themselves, each other, and preferences. All of these questions comprised the final profile.

5. The process was tiring—tiring to think about and tiring to finish.

They marched forward, and because of all the pressure, it took another six months to complete their paperwork. Just as they were putting the final touches on it, they learned a young woman outside the agency had chosen them to receive her baby. Her parents were friends who were completely familiar with the situation the Lairds were in. They immediately sent this woman to the agency, and as the wheels were already in motion, it would make the process smoother. Being chosen in advance meant they did not have to complete a family photo album and a letter to the expectant parents. This also meant their fee would be cut in half because the Lairds had brought her to the agency. They finally felt as if all the pieces were falling into place and their tenacity was paying off.

During this time, they had become part of the small group my husband and I were leading. With much joy and elation, they shared with the group that they had been chosen to receive a child. Christina went to the first ultrasound with the birth mother and found out that the baby was due in mid-March. They could barely contain their excitement. Nor could any of us. We'd been praying with them for months!

On a cold, bleak Wednesday in late January, I received a call from Christina. If her number had not come up on caller ID, I would not have known it was her. There was utter silence on the phone for several seconds until I heard soft, muffled sobs. Angela (not her real name) had changed her mind and had decided to keep the child, her fourth. None of her other children were currently in her custody. Their social worker had called to break the news. I had no words. Nothing in my comfort arsenal had prepared me for that call. "I am so sorry, Christina," was all I could manage as I fought hard to be strong for her. We cried for a brief time, and then she asked if I would mind passing the word on to the rest of the group. She couldn't bear to repeat it over and over.

This is when the bulk of Christina's mourning happened. They had been so amazed by the miracle of being chosen before they were through the entire process. Given how they had come to know God had sent them to that agency, they had been convinced all their work had been for this very reason. They had painted the nursery, and Michael's mom had driven up from Texas with a car loaded full of baby furniture and items.

Michael struggled more with the fact that Angela was going to keep the baby than he did when they found out they would not be able to have their own child. He drove to the church that same night, keeping his commitment to the youth group. He felt as if he were driving through a rain shower, but he soon realized this feeling had nothing to do with what was hitting the windshield. His tears blanketed his face. He called our pastor. He had no idea what to do with everything. It took several weeks for him to come to grips with it all. He still thinks about the fifteen-month-old girl who now would be pitter-pattering down the hallways of their home. His struggle stems in part from the fact that they see this little girl and her mom around town. They hear about the bad choices her mom continues to make. He knows how different this child's life would have been with them.

"It's not just a matter of getting your home ready," Michael said. "You also ready your heart. You can't hold back or reserve part of your heart until you get the child. You can't hold the thoughts and emotions at bay while you wait for the birth to happen." As a matter of fact, he told me everything was accelerated because they only had four months to prepare for her.

They had been told a fall-through adoption is similar in emotional experience to having a miscarriage. You want that baby. You have prepared your heart and home for that baby, and you love the child already. And then the child is gone along with all the hopes and dreams you had for that child. The difference in this case is that they had spent time cultivating a relationship with the birth mother, anticipating a lifelong relationship with her. The child is not gone. In fact, they knew they would see her every now and then. Additionally, they knew the grandparents of this child, and they were friends with her sister and family. They had every intention of keeping the child in contact with all those family members.

It took about a month for the emotional trauma to subside before they could continue the remainder of their paperwork. Even though they still struggled with the experience, they knew they had to finish the process, or they would never get a child. In April 2010, they were approved by the private agency in the Infant Adoption Program.

They began making payments for the adoption service and waiting. That waiting is by far the most difficult aspect.

While they were waiting in the summer of 2011, Angela and the little girl came into Christina's workplace while she was working. Christina's limbs went weak. She couldn't breathe. All she could think was this: *She was supposed to be my baby. God, really, what was the purpose of that?* She retreated to the bathroom and fell into a million pieces. She could make no sense of it.

The pain of that fall-through adoption continues in their hearts and minds. They feel as if they have lost a child. Yet they continue to pray for Angela and that beautiful curly-haired brunette girl.

Waiting, waiting, and more waiting. They have been waiting not only for a child but for so much more. As a result, pinpointing why it is so hard is difficult. One thing is certain: They tire and get frustrated as well-meaning person after well-meaning person tells them they understand, even as toddlers cling to the person's leg. They don't understand. They frequently hear from others that God has His reasons. Or they tell them of "someone they know" who couldn't get pregnant but as soon as the couple adopted, they had a child of their own. In fact, Christina told me she does not want that to be true for her because it not only raises the hopes of the barren womb but also devalues the life of the adopted child, as if it's not as great a joy or miracle.

As is the case with every woman I have spoken to, Christina does not want people to withhold their happiness or joy over a baby. She wants to celebrate and love that baby. She also does not want to be excluded from their lives because she does not have one. Please hear her heart and mine on this point: exclusion only exacerbates the situation. You may think you are helping, but honestly, you are not.

Looking ahead, they hope to go through the process again, even as they wait. They have no regrets.

When asked if they have advice for others in a similar situation, Michael said that while it is hard not to be self-consumed, it is important to realize that God is using the situation for a purpose in your life. "Don't turn so inward that you cannot serve, love, and help those around you. You have to work on keeping an outward focus and not let the situation rule your life, or it renders you unable to serve where He has put you. Deal with the pain as best you can. Let God do what He needs to do and keep your eyes open to what He's doing. Sometimes it's better to say nothing. Don't say, 'It's okay. God has a plan.' While those things are true, they don't always provide comfort." I wholeheartedly agree.

For Christina, the spring of 2011 was the first time she had fully allowed herself to truly mourn not having her own child. Mother's Day of that year was incredibly difficult for her. She wept through the service. God has shown her several things: Don't be ashamed of your pain. Don't wear it on your sleeve, and you shouldn't want everyone to feel sorry for you. At the same time, you must experience it. Don't deny it exists. It might not hurt forever, but it will for a while. Maybe a long while. And it will always be sad, but it is not the end of what God has for her … or you … or me.

Michael and Christina have a unique situation. They are surrounded by friends who are childless. Some have adopted. Some are still in the struggling process. Some have been through the process and have an answer, and some have no answers. They feel supported and loved through the situation. They realize not everyone has that blessing in their lives.

As our interview time came to a close, Christina remarked, "Well, I hate that our chapter is going to end with no resolution but to wait." I assured her that their waiting process would be of great hope to someone else out there who is also waiting. It will help them know they are not alone and their situation is normal.

And that was how I honestly intended to end this chapter in August 2011, for that was truly where their road had paused.

But remember how I told you I was nearly jumping out of my skin as I wrote this chapter? It is my great privilege to update Michael and Christina's journey as it stands in November 2011.

In early November, Michael stopped by our house. He was delivering cupcakes! While I was having lunch with him and Christina the week prior, I discovered that she made amazing pumpkin cupcakes and Steve loves pumpkin. So she baked some and sent them our way. While it seems odd for this to make the story, I share it now to give you insight into the heart of this amazing couple and show you what servants they are. During that visit, Michael shared with us that they had been contacted by the agency, asking if it would be okay if the staff submitted their name to a young eighteen-year-old woman due to have a child by Thanksgiving. Normally, they did not seek approval to submit profiles; however, alcohol had been consumed early in the pregnancy, and they wanted to let a prospective parent know that this consumption had happened. They enthusiastically agreed. On Tuesday, November 8, 2011, they received the news they had waited so long to hear. They had been chosen to be the parents of a little boy!

Christina could barely contain herself when she called me that night. I readily agreed when she asked me to call a list of people, and I eagerly shared their joyous news. That Friday, November 11, 2011, they headed to a town about four hours away to meet this young woman. They fell in love with her immediately. How could they not? She was sweet and kind, and she was giving them one of the greatest gifts of their lives. They returned that night, their minds reeling at the pace of everything that was happening.

The next morning, they received a call telling them that the baby had been born! They jumped in the car and headed back, secure in the knowledge they would be returning in a few days as new parents to a beautiful baby boy. Yet their prayer request was all about the birth mother. They asked their friends to pray for the emotional toll this could take on her and that they would be able to love and support her in this decision. They also desire to make her as much a part of the baby's life as she wants to be.

On Tuesday, November 15, 2011, the relinquishment papers were signed, and in May 2012, the adoption will be final. You will never meet two more ecstatic people.

It is my honor to now introduce you to Jack, the embodiment of the grace of God, the fulfillment of the hopes and promises of God. He is loved, deeply wanted, long-awaited, and a beautiful end to this chapter in the life of Michael and Christina—for now anyway. They are already planning to enter the process again.

I love him already. I am as crazy about this boy as I am about his parents.

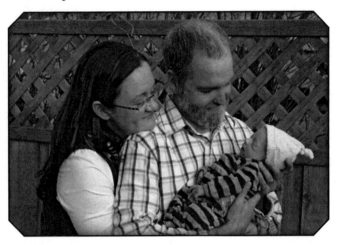

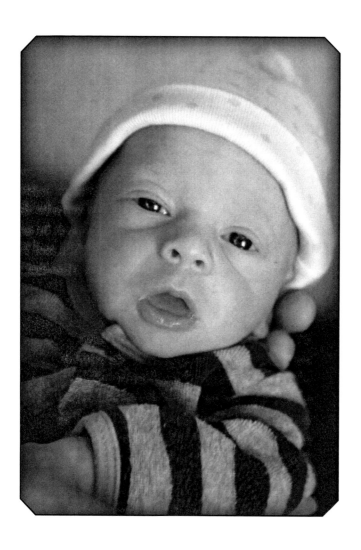

Chapter 5: When Our Choices Are Not God's

It is with great difficulty and after much prayer and consultation that I write this chapter. The subject matter is difficult. It was never God's desire for us to make the choice you'll read about in this chapter. Yet even in our sinful choices, God's redemption is fully available, and He longs to free us from the chains that bind us. Abortion is no different.

> NOTE: The names in this chapter have been changed at the request of the woman who has graciously allowed me to tell her story. This was not out of shame but rather to protect the many people involved and to ensure the spotlight and glory remain on God and not on the individual.

She is free. Even uttering those words brings tears to her eyes and some sorrow to her heart. Yes, she is free in Christ, and though she has known years of bondage, Kate understands freedom like few others.

It was 2009, and I watched a video announcement at church in sheer disbelief. What I didn't know was that it had been filmed with great trepidation. A woman I barely knew was offering an opportunity to minister to women, men, grandparents, and siblings affected by abortion. As an outsider to her life at the time, I never would have believed the story behind this uplifting, encouraging, spirit-filled woman. God had planted a seed deep in her heart that told her it was time to use her story to provide hope and help others.

Kate grew up hearing about God and attending church. She feels very blessed to have been raised in a Christian family where she was never without the love of her parents, siblings, and extended family. She fondly recalls the love and laughter that accompanied growing up in a large family surrounded by cousins, aunts, and uncles.

By age eleven, Kate had been molested twice by two different men she was familiar with through her childhood friends. One was the stepdad of one of these friends. This molestation and lost innocence caused her to develop a root of shame early on. Prior to this, she was a sweet, innocent little girl. In retrospect, she grieves for that little girl, for that young woman. It is even more grievous when she recalls that child is her. This road she has walked has given her great compassion and discernment for women and girls in similar situations.

With the prompting of her parents before the age of thirteen, Kate went through the motions of coming to Christ. She knew it was the right thing to do, so she went forward with a friend who cried at her own conversion, but she doesn't feel she truly accepted Christ at that age. There was no fruit, no growth, and no assurance of salvation. At age fifteen, she began to experiment with drugs and alcohol, and by age sixteen, she began to lead a life of sexual promiscuity, looking for love in all the wrong places. Desires that God had never intended for children of such young age had been awakened. At age eighteen, evidence pointed to the lifestyle she was living—the partying, boyfriends and alcohol. It shattered the façade that she was sweet and innocent. With great agony, Kate recalls her mother being devastated when she learned the truth about her partying lifestyle, and she remembers the disappointment in herself as well.

Kate went on to graduate from high school, although by her own admission, it was a close call. Classroom settings and keeping focused seemed difficult for her, as the shame buried deep within her led to feelings of insecurity, and she doubted her intellectual ability. The only thing she ever wanted to be as a child was a wife and mother. Her mom encouraged her to go to college for the experience if nothing else, but it was never her own desire. Nevertheless, she started a trade school in another city, but her reasoning was to get away from home and the constant reminders of shame and guilt. She didn't have to face the disappointment of her parents. Eventually, Kate quit school altogether and got random jobs.

In 1981, Kate was twenty-one, and she had been dating a young man, Chad, off and on for three years. She soon found herself pregnant and unwed. She chose not to tell her boyfriend she was pregnant, and she didn't tell anyone else either. She went to a clinic for a pregnancy test that confirmed her biggest fear. She was overcome with all the ways this would affect those around her. It would bring shame to her family. Her boyfriend would feel obligated to marry her, and she did not want to bring a baby into her lifestyle. She was drinking and doing recreational drugs and tried to rationalize all the reasons she should not have this child. It was not the way it was supposed to be.

Kate remembered a young woman she had met previously who had shared with her that she'd had two abortions. She went to her for help and advice. She did not want to tell anyone, but because she would be unable to drive herself home from the doctor, she confided in her friend Terri. Kate has very little memory of the procedure other than hearing a loud noise and closing her eyes as tightly as she could, desperately trying to block out the experience.

Chad was a good, hard-working young man who loved her, but inside where Kate was alone with her emotions and secret, she felt she was not worth much, that no one else would ever love her as Chad did. Yet she also knew if she told him about the baby, it would break his heart, so she kept the abortion secret. Kate further rationalized by assuring herself she and Chad would eventually have a child at some point in their marriage and that birth would make up for the decision to abort her first baby. It would lessen the pain.

In 1982, Kate and Chad married. A short year later, at age twenty-four, she lost her mom very suddenly to cancer.

She went to her grave, never knowing Kate had been molested or had undergone an abortion. As it turns out, adoption had played a big role in her extended family because two of her siblings had adopted children. She didn't want to tell them because she felt she would be thought of as a monster.

Kate kept this secret for a long time but eventually confided in one of her sisters, swearing her to secrecy. She had not intended to share this when she did, but there came a time when her older sister, Kristy, mentioned a friend of hers having an abortion, and as she spoke, she noticed a strange look come over Kate's face. Kristy asked her if she'd had an abortion, which caused Kate to break her silence and confide in her that yes, it was true. Despite their nine-year difference, these two sisters had always been extremely close. That conversation is what God used to break that root of shame along with some other pressing questions Kristy eventually came to ask Kate, specifically concerning her salvation.

Kate and Chad continued the party lifestyle they had always lived. About five years into the marriage, she grew weary of their union, which had seemingly become one big party to her. Chad began to notice she wasn't the same person. She was not the fun-loving wife he had married. Her heart was changing. As he stood in the kitchen one day, he said, "You're going to leave me, aren't you?" After much begging for the lifestyle to stop and for them to go to counseling and church, she took matters into her own hands and left. She had a good job and eventually found an apartment in a nearby town. She was already experiencing physical ailments, and then she was hospitalized.

They stayed married for another three years, seeing each other off and on, and at one point, they did reconcile briefly. She did not want to be the one to file for the divorce. She knew her vows were solemn. In the midst of this time at age twenty-eight, she hit a wall and realized she desperately needed a savior. God got her attention in many ways that opened her eyes to this fact. Kate knew something was very wrong physically. She was bleeding internally, and her soul was filled with shame and regret. Because she fully believed the promise of Romans 10:9, she prayed to receive Christ in her apartment at that moment. She couldn't wait to go to church that weekend. She was on fire and could not wait for everyone to see her changed heart. Eventually, Chad began to see someone else, and Kate found herself served with divorce papers. She was thirty years old.

For a few years, she had one foot in the church and one in the world. She had moved into what she refers to as the "elite" world of partying. She became a "career woman who had been divorced," and nine years later, she was still keeping her secret. Ultimately, this secret became too much for her to keep, and during one of her down times with her illness, she stayed with her brother, Bill, and his wife. She began to weep and told him she'd had an abortion. After years of fearing she would be alienated by her family, she was relieved at the care and concern she was shown. Bill had a four-year-old daughter who was named after her, and they shared a room while Kate was staying with them and being cared for by them. The night after she had finally shared her secret with her brother, that beautiful little girl she loved so much nestled next to her. For the first time since the abortion, she felt hope and love. She sensed the power of God through that innocent child lying next to her in that bed. The tears fell that night as she felt a true mother-child bond with her little niece. They suddenly shared so much more than a name. Kate knew healing would eventually come. Recognizing she was a new creation in Christ, she clung tightly to 2 Corinthians 5:17. There was no doubt of the full redemption God had poured onto her and the forgiveness she need only to accept.

Kate moved on with her life but found she avoided friends with babies whenever she could help it. She never desired to hold a baby for fear of the emotions it could trigger. She did not want to think about the child she did not have. She never told the father. Chad remarried, and together, he and his second wife had a son.

As time passed, Kate began attending church regularly and pursued a relationship with Christ. Having encountered wolves in sheep's clothing, she determined to pursue Christ first and Christ alone. It was time for her to leave the dating world behind and get to know Jesus as she never had before. Kate met the single adult leader and began to attend events for single people her age, not as a means to meet someone but to be encouraged to grow in her faith with others in a similar stage of life. Additionally, she was able to manage her illness off and on for eleven years.

As time passed, however, Kate's physical health began to decline. God placed godly people in her life that helped her along the way. One of them was a man by the name of Joe. He had all the qualifications of a good husband, but in her own mind, she was damaged goods. She was divorced. She had had an abortion, and she was sick.

They began a friendship with no thoughts of any further relationship. As a matter of fact, Kate had told the Lord that if He wanted her to be in a relationship, He would have to bring a man who loved Him first and would love her as Christ loved the church. If not, she was content being a bride of Christ.

What she and Joe did not know was that God was weaving their lives together. They began dating, discussed her divorce, searched the Scriptures, and talked about marriage. Kate had no intention of purposely hiding her abortion from him, but she did not necessarily see a need to tell him outright.

While they were out canoeing one day, Joe began asking Kate random questions. What she thought was just a fun, relaxing day, he was using intentionally to ask her very pointed questions. One of those questions was, "How do you feel about abortion?"

Kate replied, "Well, I don't agree with it." As a child of Christ, God had changed her entire attitude about the issue, and she knew the sinfulness of it now.

As a follow-up question, for reasons unknown even to him, he asked, "Have you ever had one?"

A rush of shame, guilt and sorrow enveloped her. Panic seized her. She immediately denied it.

They returned to her townhouse for dinner, and as they sat down, Kate began weeping and sobbing. Surprised and dismayed, Joe asked what was wrong. She asked, "Do you remember the question you asked me on the lake?" He had asked her so many questions that day he had no idea which she was referring to exactly.

For the first time, she said the word out loud—abortion. She asked, "Remember when you asked if I had had an abortion? I lied to you. I have had an abortion." The tears kept coming. Joe put his arm around her, and with great compassion, he reminded her that Christ had forgiven her and she did not have to live in condemnation any longer. (See Romans 8:1.) He was deeply concerned that she understood what forgiveness meant. She was the woman at the well, and he was speaking words of Christ. She knew she had been forgiven by Christ for all her sins, but she could not forgive herself. For years, she had asked herself, "How could a woman murder her own baby?" She was horrified by her actions. She was a horrible monster, and abortion was an unpardonable sin to her.

They fell to their knees, and as Kate cried, Joe told her to simply talk to God about it. Although she had confessed that before and knew she had been forgiven, she asked God to help her forgive herself, to make the head and heart connect. God answered that prayer. Kate began on a journey, and God is using that part of her past to minister to other women. Not just to women but also to men, grandparents, siblings, children, other family and friends who have been affected by abortion.

At last, Kate understood that her secret could not be kept secret forever. She was not an island. Her sin had affected others, and it had injured them.

Kate has never had another pregnancy. She has never given birth to a child. Yet she is freer at fifty-one than ever before in her life. After seasons of longing for a child, she is full and complete in her life. She and Joe have committed their lives to serving God in their church and community. Children are everywhere in her life, and each one is a constant reminder of God's amazing mercy and grace.

Kate's story is one of hope and redemption. Her sin of abortion has been fully forgiven, and she knows without a doubt that, like Esther, her story is for such a time as this. In a culture where abortion is frequent, voices like hers are needed. While God does not approve of our sin, He does offer full and complete forgiveness and healing. She has been given an enormous opportunity.

Does she still think about that baby? Absolutely! She has wondered throughout the years about how that person, who would now be a thirty-year-old, would look, what job he or she would have, and many other things. But she no longer wonders through the lenses of shame and guilt. She takes comfort in knowing her child has been with Christ this entire time. She knows their reunion is yet to come.

And while she waits, Kate sings the praises of the One who redeemed her life from the pit. She dances beautifully before the Lord. Her eyes well with tears as she recites one of her favorite passages of Scripture (Psalm 103:1–4):

> Praise the Lord O my soul;
> All my innermost being, praise his Holy Name.
> Praise the Lord O my soul and forget not all His benefits.
> Who forgives all your sins and heals all your diseases,
> Who redeems your life from the pit and crowns you with love and compassion.

Chapter 6: The Stigma …
or Blessing?

I TRUST BY NOW YOU'VE been encouraged by the stories in the previous chapters. I'd like to spend a little bit of time proving that while children are a beautiful gift from God, not having a child doesn't mean a person is of less value. There is frequently a stigma attached to the childless, but separating fact from emotion is of great value in the process of acceptance.

Have you ever listened to the many ways people introduce themselves? Over the years, I've begun to pay attention to this, probably because I've been unbelievably sensitive about it. Nevertheless, I have noticed. Many times women introduce themselves as the wife of someone, the mother of someone, or by the position they hold in their professional life. It almost seems as if there is no identity outside of a job title, children, or a husband. Don't get me wrong. I have fallen into this trap time and time again. I have delighted in the career titles I've earned over the years. Granted, these things make us who we are, but they are not the sole identifiers. I heard about a business meeting where the organizer had the attendees circulate and meet each other. The only criterion was that they could not mention their occupation in their conversation. As you might imagine, the first several minutes were very quiet and somewhat awkward. It was definitely outside the norm to find a different way to identify oneself, particularly in that business setting. These participants had no idea how to begin a conversation.

Several years ago, I read a quote by Dr. William H. Thomas, a geriatric specialist. He has noted that babies begin life by *being*. As we approach adulthood, the emphasis shifts to achievement or success. Then, as we grow older still and our energy fades, we must refocus on existing. "Elderhood brings us full circle," Thomas says, "to a life that favors *being* over *doing*. This is a gift of great value."

How true this is! Our identity shifts from what is valued in us to what we do or to whom we belong only to return to the realization that who we are in Christ provides our true value and is all that really matters.

I have a friend who always identified herself as the mother of her children or the wife of her husband. Never once in the first six years I knew her did she ever identify herself by something she enjoyed doing or a particular aspect of her personality. It was as if she had no uniqueness outside her immediate family or any purpose to fulfill just by the nature of being her. I am not saying that she shouldn't revel in being a wife and mother; however, I always knew God had a purpose that only she could fulfill, and it was not because she was married or she had children. Since that time and as her children have grown and moved out of the house, she has obtained employment outside the home and has become involved in some ladies' ministries in her church. It has been exciting to watch her blossom and hear her talk about herself and her life outside her family every once in a while. I love it when she tells me what God is doing in her life and how she is growing and maturing in her faith. It has nothing to do with her children or her husband but rather who she is in Christ. I cannot get over how exciting that is to me.

I have often wondered why women feel the need to identify themselves by who they married or to whom they gave birth, and I think I finally tripped across a possible answer. There is a stigma tied to women who cannot have or do not want children, women who choose not to marry or opt for a vocation as homemaker rather than one in corporate America. Since ancient times, women have been defined by who they have married or to whom they have given birth. Without a husband or children, many considered them to be lesser women, outcasts, and they were sentenced to a life of destitution. To a certain, lesser degree, this holds true today. It is evidenced by the questions posed to the woman who has no child. What is wrong with you? Why wouldn't you want a child? These questions are emotionally charged, causing us to feel inferior. We may be more sophisticated in the words we say or how we approach the situation, but for those of us on the childless side, we feel it just the same. Of one thing I am convinced, barrenness knows no bounds. It is no respecter of gender, race, culture, or creed.

While it is important to embrace the roles God has placed us in, ranging from wife to mother or grandmother, it is even more important to fulfill what I call the "kingdom role." God has a transcendent purpose for each and every one of us. If that were not true, we would not be here. Evidence of this is found in Psalm 139, which is one of my favorite chapters in the Bible. Write verse 16 of this chapter below.

_____

_____

_____

_____

Our days are ordained by none other than God Himself. Nowhere in that verse or the surrounding verses does it say this applies only to mothers. That tells me God has made certain women to be mothers or wives and others not. But we all have a role to fulfill in our ordained days. None of them are lesser jobs, just different.

Let's look for a minute at 1 Corinthians 7. I encourage you to read it in its entirety, but what I want to pull out is a principle Paul discusses. This chapter is focused on marriage relationships; however, I believe we can apply the principle to the childless as well. What does verse 7 say?

_____

_____

_____

Paul considered his singleness a gift from God! Can we not apply that same principle and those same words to the childless? God has chosen some to receive the gift of being childless so they can focus their energy on ministry for Him. The truth is that children, while wonderful on so many levels, tie the parents to a lifetime commitment. Those without children are free to serve God in ways those with children never can. Let's read 1 Corinthians 7:32. What does this verse say?

_____

_____

_____

_____

Again, Paul relates this sentiment to being unmarried versus married, but the same principle applies. Women without children are *free* from the concerns that naturally go with being a mother. They can now turn their entire focus to the Lord's affairs and how to please Him. I don't know about you, but as a woman who has never given birth, this gives me great encouragement.

One of the biggest mistakes we make is trying to find our value in something other than Christ. The world places our identity in children, spouses, money, physical appearance, power, prestige, athleticism, and intelligence. While there is value in *being* a mother or a wife, that is not the *source of* our value. Who we are in Christ is what *makes* us valuable. Dear reader, we are precious to God, no matter how many children we bear or don't. God values all His children. Consider the following verses:

> I Peter 2:4
> As you come to Him, the living Stone—
> rejected by men but chosen by God and

precious to him – you also, like living
stones, are being built into a spiritual house
to be a holy priesthood, offering spiritual
sacrifices acceptable to God through Jesus
Christ.

Luke 12:24
Consider the ravens; they do not sow or
reap, they have no storeroom or barn; yet
God feeds them. And how much more
valuable you are than the birds!

Genesis 1:31
God saw all that He had made, and it was
very good (emphasis mine).

Psalm 8:3–5
When I consider your heavens the work of
your fingers, the moon and the stars which
you have set in place, what is man that you
are mindful of him, the son of man that you
care for him? You made him a little lower
than the heavenly beings and crowned him
with glory and honor.

Psalm 113:5–9
Who is like the Lord our God, the One who
sits enthroned on high, who stoops down
to look on the heavens and the earth? He
raises the poor from the dust and lifts the
needy from the ash heap; he seats them with

princes, with the princes of their people. He
settles the barren woman in her home as a
happy mother of children. Praise the Lord.

I think my favorite of these passages is the last one, Psalm
113:5–9, because it is evidence that God does not elevate
His children based on their occupation, their wealth,
and their social status, and He certainly does not show
favoritism because some have children. He exalts the
unlikely, raises up the peasant, and uses the barren woman
to her full potential in Him.

So is the inability to have children a stigma and curse
or a blessing? After I researched God's word, I have to
conclude that it is as much of a blessing as having children
is. It could be a blessing to a child you are about to adopt,
or it could be a blessing to the calling you have in God's
work. We cannot allow other people in our lives or the
cultures in which we live determine that we are cursed.
God is very clear that until He comes again or takes us
home, we do have a purpose—children or not.

The Bible has something to say about anything and
everything that happens in our lives. It should come
as no surprise that it has something to say about being
barren and provides us with some examples of women who
experienced this very thing.

I think it is important to note that regardless of whether or
not God brought children into the lives of these women,
the lessons are in their journey, their cries to God, His
answers, and their responses. Please do not get caught up,

as I did initially, in the fact that God did eventually bless these women with children. If you do, you will miss the point of their example and the realizations they had of God's role in their lives. While the end result is of value to God and to us, the true mark of our growth comes in our journey and how we respond to God as we make the journey. Do we obey or not? Frequently, the outcome is deeply impacted by the steps of faith we take, and the end result simply marks the completion of a great work God did in and through us.

Chapter 7: They Got It Right! The Stories of Hannah and Elizabeth

Hannah

THE STORY OF HANNAH IS told in 1 Samuel 1 and 2. Let's lay some ground work to help you get a complete understanding on the woman named Hannah. Read these two chapters.

Who was Hannah married to (1:1)?_____

_____

_____

What unusual characteristic marked their marriage (1:2)?

_____

_____

I won't go into great detail to discuss the cultural acceptance of multiple wives in that time, but I cannot let it pass without saying that prevalence in society does not mean permission from God. Let me prove this to you specifically regarding this issue. Read Matthew 19:4–6 below:

"Haven't you read," he replied, "that at the beginning the Creator made them male and female and said, "For this reason a man will leave his father and mother and be united to his wife, and the two will become one flesh?" So they are no longer two, but one. Therefore what God has joined together, let man not separate."

According to these verses, who is to be married?_____

_____

How many are to be married?_____

_____

The reason it is so important to note that this marriage is outside of God's design is because it gives us insight to the relationship of these two women. Hannah's feelings of insecurity are further exacerbated by something else we learn in 1 Samuel 1:2.

What did Peninnah have that Hannah did not?_____

_____

How did Elkanah try to compensate for Hannah's grief (1:5)?_____

Why did he do this?_____

_____

_____

Who had closed Hannah's womb?_____

_____

The Bible does not say whether or not Hannah realized how much Elkanah loved her, but it is obvious to anyone who reads these verses how much he loved her. It must not have had anything to do with her ability to bear children because she did not have any. Nevertheless, she was completely consumed with sorrow over being barren. I can relate to her in this regard.

To make matters worse, this second wife would not leave Hannah alone. What did her "rival," as the NIV states it, do to her in verse 6?_____

_____

_____

Why did she do this?_____

_____

_____

How long did this go on (v7)?_____

_____

This constant anguish eventually had physical effects on Hannah as well. She wept and wouldn't eat. This part of the story breaks my heart. As if it were not bad enough that Hannah was an emotional wreck, this other woman in her marriage was fruitful and had children. She tormented Hannah. Elkanah tried desperately to comfort her to no avail (verse 8). With the exception of the two-wife thing, it is almost as if I am reading my own story. Steve, along with many others, tried greatly to console me. I would have none of it. I was taunted with insensitive comments, such as, "What is wrong with you that you don't have kids?" Like Hannah, I wept bitterly year after year after year.

But unlike Hannah, I did not respond very well. According to 1 Samuel 1:10–11, what did Hannah do?

_____

_____

_____

It goes on in verse 15 to say she poured out her soul to the Lord. If only I had read this story twelve years ago! In spite of everything going on in her life—her closed womb and family turmoil—Hannah never lost sight of God. Here in the midst of her sorrow and despair, she recognized that God was the answer. She recognized His holiness and reached out to Him for healing.

I do not want to pretend the rest of the story doesn't exist because that would do a severe injustice to the Scriptures. God answered Hannah's prayer that day, and Samuel was born to her. She kept her commitment to God and dedicated him to a lifetime of service to God just as she vowed in 1 Samuel 1:11. Samuel grew up to be one of the greatest judges in Israel. Please do not get stuck here because the truth is that God may never answer your prayer for a child. He did not for me either. The most important thing in this story is that Hannah did not reject God or turn from Him. As a matter of fact, she ran straight to Him. The first ten verses of 1 Samuel 2 record Hannah's prayer of joy to the Lord. Her journey and response were right.

Elizabeth

Let's take a look at a second story highlighting a great response to barrenness. This story features none other than Elizabeth, the cousin of Mary, the mother of Jesus.

This narrative is found in Luke chapter 1. The focus verses are five through seven.

Who was Elizabeth married to?_____

_____

What was his occupation?_____

_____

What was his lineage?_____

_____

What was Elizabeth's lineage?_____

_____

What do we learn of their spiritual life in verse 6?_____

_____

_____

_____

Why did they not have children?_____

_____

_____

What else do we learn about Zechariah and Elizabeth in verse 7?_____

_____

_____

_____

Being from the lineage of Aaron meant Zechariah and Elizabeth were to minister before the Lord in the temple. (See Exodus 28.) Essentially, they were in full-time ministry. Yet their lives were not picture perfect. They had struggles, heartaches, and unmet desires just like I do and just like you do. I am reminded of my mom's words so many years ago. Life is not fair. None of us are exempt from struggle because of our heritage, our occupation, our spouse, having children, or anything else. In fact, talk to any parent you meet, and they will likely tell you how much their struggles and heartaches have increased.

While it may not seem like much at first glance, I glean so much out of these verses about the character and relationship of Elizabeth and Zechariah. The fact that they were well along in years makes me believe they had been married for quite some time. Their relationship was not at all based on having children. The most important thing, however, is that they were both upright and followed God's commands. Elizabeth did not wallow in self-pity, and she did not choose to believe she was of no value to God without a family. It must have been extremely difficult for her to live in those times when she had never given birth. She continued to serve God and pursued a relationship with him while she maintained what I believe was an amazing relationship with her husband. Now that's a right response!

Let's conclude this portion by noting who this child was. Read Luke 1:57–80.

What did Elizabeth and Zechariah name the baby?_____

_____

What was his calling or purpose? (See verse 76.)_____

_____

What did Jesus say about him in Matthew 11:11?_____

_____

While this chapter was not intended to be about John the Baptist, I could not help asking these past few questions. This child of elderly, formerly barren parents had an amazing life and purpose in the time of Christ. Incidentally, Scripture and historical texts do not note if John was married or if he had children of his own. Yet he had an incredible, well-lived life, and he fulfilled his purpose before God called him home (see Mark 6:17–29).

Chapter 8: Not Quite Right! The Stories of Rachel and Sarah

IN CONTRAST TO THE PREVIOUS chapter, I want to take a look at a couple of responses that were very different from Hannah and Elizabeth.

Rachel

The story of Rachel is told in Genesis 29–35, but my main focus concerns chapter 30. Before we get to this chapter, let's establish some groundwork about this family.

Read Genesis 25:19–26 and answer the following questions:

Who are the parents of Jacob?_____

_____

What was noteworthy about the birth of Jacob?_____

_____

While I'm not specifically focusing on Rebekah, the mother of Jacob and Esau, I would like you to take in what is important enough to be noted in the verse 21.

What was true of Rebekah?_____

_____

What did Isaac do about this problem?_____

_____

I love the idea of a man praying for his wife, particularly about her barrenness. Can you imagine how heartbroken Rebekah must have been and how this must have deeply affected Isaac? What a tender thing for him to do—intercede on her behalf to God. In this case, God responded with not one but two babies—twins, one a skillful hunter and one a quiet man. Simply amazing.

For the record, according to Genesis 32:27–28, who did Jacob become?_____

_____

Young Jacob, who is later renamed Israel, becomes the father of the twelve tribes of Israel. In Genesis 29 and 30, we read the account of the family Jacob has, and we see another occurrence of multiple wives. As with Hannah, this story also records the women at odds, pitted against each other, vying for the attention and affections of their shared husband.

Read Genesis 29:15–30:24.

Why is Jacob working for Laban?_____

_____

Note what Scripture says about Leah and Rachel in 29:15–18:

How did Laban deceive Jacob?_____

_____

_____

_____

What reason did he give for doing this?_____

_____

_____

_____

What did Laban require of Jacob to get Rachel?_____

_____

Of the two, which one was Jacob's favorite?_____

_____

When God saw Leah was not loved, what did He do?_

_____

_____

What is Leah trying to achieve in verses 31-35?_____

_____

_____

_____

In Genesis 30:1, what is Rachel's response?_____

_____

According to verse 2, who kept Rachel from having children?_____

This situation is a mess. Let's talk about it for a few minutes. Both Laban and Jacob have put these women in a no-win situation. By marrying off both daughters, Laban's responsibility was complete. He had no further worries about caring for his daughters. But he set them up for a life of turmoil. Jacob furthered this turmoil by favoring one greatly over the other. I'm sure this was a natural response. He deeply loved Rachel. He had always loved Rachel. The evidence of this is found in the fact that he was willing to work seven years for her and further proven when he worked fourteen for her. In great sadness, chapter 29 ends with Leah trying to win Jacob's affections by having not only child after child but son after son. Having a son in biblical times caused a woman to be highly praised. In verse 32, she remarked, "Surely my husband will love me now." Then in verse 34, we read Leah saying, "At last my husband will become attached to me." This is heart-wrenching. Leah was tying her value in life to how Jacob felt about her and to the quantity of children she could bear rather than who God had created her to be. But read a gem in Genesis 29:35.

What is Leah's response finally?_____
_____

Leah grasped the truth, at least momentarily. We'll see her fall back a bit in chapter 30, but for that season, she praised the Lord.

As I am sure you noted above, chapter 30 opens with Rachel having a fit of jealousy. She equated Jacob's love for her with the quantity of children she could provide to him and failed to recognize the complete devotion he must have had to her. This reaction didn't bode well for her, as it only made Jacob angry. Rachel then did something that I cannot even comprehend—she gave her maidservant to her husband to start a family! Just what this story needed was another woman thrown into the mix. This strategy seemingly worked for Rachel, as Bilhah conceived and gave birth to two sons, but there is great sadness in Rachel's response.

What is her response in 30:8?_____

_____

_____

_____

It appears that for Rachel, the competition with Leah was of greater importance than actually having and loving children. For her, barrenness meant she did not have Jacob's love, and so she tried to earn it another way. Isn't that exactly like us? Rachel placed her entire self-worth on whether or not she had children. She never stopped to think that God loved her anyway, as did Jacob, and that her barrenness was not the identifier of who she was. It was not about winning or losing but relationships.

Before we move on, let's summarize the rest of this portion of Scripture. Leah stopped having children and did exactly as Rachel had. She gave her maidservant to Jacob. In case you lost count (and that would be easy to do), we now have four women competing for the affections of one man. The boys these maidservants bore were "credited" to Leah and Rachel as was customary at the time. In all, twelve sons were born to Jacob:

<u>Leah</u>: Reuben Simeon Levi Judah Issachar Zebulun	<u>Rachel</u>: Joseph Benjamin
<u>Zilpah</u> (Leah's maidservant): Gad Asher	<u>Bilhah</u> (Rachel's maidservant): Dan Naphtali

There were plenty of blessings in this story, but there were plenty of heartaches and wrong responses as well. I believe Rachel's journey and response were not at all what God wanted to see from her. As a matter of fact, she only further complicated the familial relationship with her sister. This dysfunctional family dynamic continued in the lives of the children born to these women and Jacob. Anger, resentment, and jealousy became commonplace among these sons, and they came by it naturally. If you need evidence as to whether the decisions you make matter or impact those around you, this story definitely provides confirmation for you.

Sarah

The second story I want to highlight is that of Sarah, which is found in Genesis 11–25, but I am going to center this section on the parts of the story in chapters 15, 16, and 18. To avoid confusion, in chapter 15, you'll see the name "Sarai," and this is the same person as "Sarah" in chapter 18. Likewise, the same is true with "Abram" and "Abraham." In Genesis 17:15 and 17:5, God changed their names. For sake of continuity, I will refer to them solely as Sarah and Abraham.

According to Genesis 15:3, what was the reason Abraham had no children?_____

_____

_____

In this same chapter, God promised not just an heir to Abraham but so many he would not be able to count them (verse 5). Yet the timing does not seem acceptable to Sarah because in chapter 16, we read an account eerily similar to what we just studied in the lives of Rachel and Leah.

Read Genesis 16:1–6.

What did Sarah do in verse 2?_____

_____

What was the result in verse 4?_____

_____

How did Hagar respond to her mistress (v4)?

_____

Who did Sarah blame for this?_____

_____

What was Abraham's response to Sarah?_____

_____

_____

_____

What action did Sarah take?_____

_____

Just as we have the same response from Sarah as we did from Rachel, we also have the same result. Jealousy emerged. Hagar despised her mistress, and Sarah mistreated her so badly it caused Hagar to flee into the desert. Heartache abounded in this story all because of wrong responses.

Let's fast forward to Genesis 18. In this chapter, we see Abraham getting three visitors, one of whom was the Lord. Once again, we see the promise of God in verse 10: "Then the Lord said, 'I will surely return to you about this time next year, and Sarah your wife will have a son.'"

What was Sarah's response in verse 12? She laughed. Not only did she laugh, but she lied when confronted about it (verse 15). Scripture goes on to tell us that once Isaac was born and weaned, Sarah insisted that Abraham send Hagar and her son away, and that was exactly what happened (Genesis 21:10).

What I want you to understand in the story of these two women is that their journeys and responses were sinful and carried harsh consequences. Both of them suffered from jealousy brought on entirely by their own decisions. They also strained relationships with their family, maidservants, and husbands. That does not mean God did not make good of these situations. He did. But the consequence in the meantime for Rachel and Leah was a marred relationship. For Hagar and Sarah, it meant the end of a relationship and the separation of father and son. The children of these unions were also victims of the decisions of their mothers.

Just as the responses of Hannah, Elizabeth, Rachel, and Sarah mattered, so do mine, and so do yours. How you choose to handle your inability to have children will affect those around you. It can lead to strained or ruined relationships, anger, jealousy, hatred, and bitterness. It can also affect the next generation, should God bless you with children of your own. Please do not take that to mean you cannot or will not experience a plethora of emotions. You absolutely will. Emotions in and of themselves are a natural part of how we are made. Jesus had emotions while on earth as a man. He experienced sorrow, frustration, and anger. He was tempted as we are, yet was without sin. The problem is not the emotion itself but what we do with it and how it is expressed.

As a final note to these chapters, you might have noticed I asked repeatedly who closed the wombs of these women, if Scripture noted it for us. I did this on purpose. If Scripture takes the time to record something, it is worthy for us to take notice. As women unable to have children, we need to understand that this is God's plan. Life and death are completely under His control. That knowledge may require you to ask even more questions about who has the ability to have a child and who does not. Whether we understand that or not, it is truth. God is in charge of life. It is not an accident or happenstance but rather part of what He has for my life and for your life. The sooner you can understand that, the easier the road will become. It is a pivotal point.

Chapter 9: The Crossroads

I'VE SPENT THE LAST COUPLE of chapters talking about barren women, their journeys, and their responses. I stated in chapter six that I believe God is more interested in our journey and response than He is in the end result, and I hope you can see through these biblical examples that this is the case. And so we are at the crossroads, the end of the book. I invite you to decide your response.

The response of our natural self looks much like my initial response and that of Sarah and Rachel. First, I pretended it did not exist. That was an effective way for me to hold up under the pain, albeit for a brief time. Soon enough, time began to pass, and the things I used to fill that ache were no longer effective. I had tried to fill my sadness in so many ways. We bought new cars, the latest technology, and more shoes and purses than I could count. I pursued, and achieved, success in the business world. I won awards and accolades. I received raises, bonuses, and promotions. We traveled to fun and exciting places. And just when those did not work, I tried to convince Steve we needed to move. In my mind, a change of venue would be new and I could focus my energy on settling in and learning about a new place. It would fill my time, my head, and my heart with enough variance that I could forget about it for a while. He never agreed and so we never moved. Soon all those things seemed empty to me as well. I could not fill the void with things. I had to confront it. Additionally, I was faced with the reality that I was getting older. Time did not stop my pain. As a matter of fact, the pain screamed so loudly in my being that I eventually had to stop pretending and face the facts. Second, I blamed God. It is so easy to do this. If we can blame someone else, anyone else, then we never have to own the truth. Even if it is not our fault, the truth is what it is, and blaming others is a weak façade that will eventually crash in around us. Third, I felt sorry for myself and took it out on everyone around me. This is playing the victim at its best. It is fascinating to note that I did not plan these steps. They all came out as a result of a natural flow in my sinful nature. Satan would have loved to keep me in bondage over this for the rest of my life and render me useless to God, so I obviously did not feel any resistance to these selfish emotions. It was not until out of the depths of the pit when I looked at God and allowed Him to pull me up that I felt any attack from Satan. And since then, I have been the target of so many attacks I cannot count them all. Once God called me to put pen and paper to my experience and impressed on my heart that so many women out there needed to hear this, the real warfare began. I have been pulled and tugged and torn to pieces again and again.

I am frequently asked, "Does it still hurt?" Without hesitation, my answer is, "Yes, it still hurts." Sometimes a lot, other times not as much, but it does still hurt. That does not mean I dwell in it every day. Wanting a child is a desire that will always be unmet for me, but it does not have to be the end *for* me or the end *of* me. It is an area Satan can use to cause me to fall flat in a heartbeat.

I must always guard against it. It can hurt and yet be okay at the same time. Let me explain because I saw this principle quite clearly a few years back. My dad passed away suddenly and unexpectedly at the age of sixty-three in 2006, much too soon for my liking. But God knew better, and He made no mistake in my dad's death. God didn't forget about my dad or look away for a minute only to turn back and discover him gone. My dad's days were ordained, and his purpose was obviously completed. I will miss him until the day of my last breath; however, I do not dwell in that pain and I have not lost hope. It hurts some days, and I am okay in that same moment.

Think of it this way: God is aware of sin and sees sin. He just cannot dwell in it because of His character and His righteousness. If He could dwell with sin, there would not have been need of a savior. But there was. That is the first key to overcoming that which seems insurmountable. I could never have done this on my own. It is Christ in me. Perhaps you have never come to that place in your life where you have acknowledged your need of Christ as savior—that is truly the starting place. Without Christ there is no hope—not in this situation or any other. 1 John 1:9 tells us that if we confess our sins, He is faithful and just to forgive our sins and cleanse us from all unrighteousness. Romans 10:13 tells us that everyone who calls on the name of the Lord will be saved. If you have never made that decision, I promise you that nothing else in your life is more important. Knowing for certain where you will spend eternity is the greatest sense of peace and security you will ever know. Then and only then can you win the battle raging in your barren womb and heart.

Another thing I am frequently asked is if the journey has been worth it or if I would do it again. The answer of "yes" is surprising even to me. This entire experience has shaken me to the core of my being in a time when I was questioning my very belief system about God and wondering if it was worth serving, giving, and devoting my entire life to Him. He removed everything from me so that I had no choice but to look directly in His face. Once that happened, there was no possible way for me to deny who God was and who He wanted me to be. I know exactly what I believe and in whom I believe. How could I come face-to-face with the God of the universe and say, "No thanks?" I couldn't, and I doubt you can either.

The journey was absolutely worth it, because He is worth it. And you are worth it too. Part of my purpose in this journey has been for you. God loves you so much, and more than anything, He wants to heal you and make you complete in Him. Won't you begin your journey to Him now? I challenge you as you turn the last page of this book to write a prayer to God, one telling Him exactly how you feel. Be honest. God can take it. Then leave it at His feet and begin to heal. Develop an accountability group to support you and pray for you. There is a light at the end of the tunnel, and that light is beckoning you to Him.

Thank you for sharing in my journey. Before I leave you with a final promise from Scripture, I want to share with you a recent victory in this lifelong, wild ride. Just two weeks ago, I did something I swore I would never do again. I hosted a baby shower. I can barely believe it myself. Remember baby Jack and his beautiful mother,

Christina, in chapter 4? They were the reason for this unprecedented event. And it was incredibly difficult but so worth it for them … and for me. That can be your reality too. One day at a time—no more, no less.

And now for a promise from Philippians 1:6: "being confident of this, that he who began a good work in you will carry it on to completion until the day of Christ Jesus."

A good work is being done, even if you don't see it or understand it. I will end with a poem I wrote in October 2003 during a time that had nothing to do with my inability to have children. But in looking over it, I believe it applies every bit as much to this journey as the one we were going through when I wrote it. I hope you draw encouragement from it.

Grace in the Face of Trials

Standing on the brink, the edge dangerously near,

I am so confused; how did I get here?

I serve and I give, study and learn.

So what went wrong? For the answer I yearn.

How is it, Lord, the children you love

can be so broken with no word from above?

The events of life left me wounded once more.

Lord, how many times till you open that door?

The guilt is great from the anger I feel;

directed at You, Lord, why won't You heal?

Is it something I've done that brought all this on?

Or is it Your will, greater glory to spawn?

Please, Lord, give me answers to heal this torn heart.

Show me Your love before I fall apart.

And, Lord, give me strength, sustain me with grace;

should no answer come, not to turn from Your face.

I pray peace for you as you make this journey. May you come to a place of acceptance and understanding. May God bless you richly as you strive to serve Him. He loves you more deeply than you can comprehend.

CPSIA information can be obtained at www.ICGtesting.com
Printed in the USA
BVOW012352100512

289908BV00005B/7/P